Disclaimer

It's important to note that I am not a medical professional or personal trainer, and the information provided should not be taken as medical advice. Before starting any exercise or nutritional program, it is recommended that you consult with a healthcare professional, especially if you have any pre-existing medical conditions or concerns. This is to ensure that you are physically able to engage in the activities that you have planned and to prevent any potential injuries or health complications. Additionally, it's important to start slowly and gradually increase the intensity and duration of your exercise routine to avoid over-exertion and to allow your body time to adjust. Furthermore, be sure to listen to your body, if you feel pain or discomfort, stop the activity and rest. Always make sure to get professional advice and guidance.

DO THE EASY FITNESS

" Weight Loss Motivation: Your Path to a Healthier You"

Do The Easy Fitness Philosophy

Exercise and Nutrition are two of the most powerful tools we have for improving our physical and mental health. Regular physical activity can help to reduce the risk of chronic diseases such as heart disease, diabetes, and obesity. It can also improve our mood, increase our energy levels, and help us to sleep better. However, despite the numerous benefits of exercise, many people struggle to find the motivation to make it a regular part of their lives. This is where Do The Easy Fitness comes in. It's about motivating yourself and others with everyday Lifestyle changes.

One key to staying motivated is to set specific, achievable goals for yourself. For example, you might set a goal to run a 5K race in the next six months, or to lose a certain amount of weight. Having a clear, measurable goal can help you to stay focused and on track. Additionally, it is essential to find an activity that you enjoy and that fits your lifestyle. Whether it be going for a walk, swimming, cycling, or joining a sports team, finding an activity that you enjoy will make it more likely that you will stick with it.

Another important factor in staying motivated is to have a support system. Having a workout partner or joining a fitness class can help to keep you accountable, and also make the exercise more fun. Also, it is important to remind yourself of the benefits of exercise, not only for the present but also for the future. Regular exercise can help to improve your overall quality of life, both now and in the long-term.

Finally, it is essential to remember that there will be setbacks and obstacles along the way. There will be days when you don't feel like exercising, sticking to your nutritional goals, or when you miss a workout. The important thing is not to let these setbacks discourage you. Instead, focus on getting back on track as soon as possible and not to give up on yourself. Remember that a healthy and active lifestyle is a lifelong commitment and it takes time, patience, and perseverance to make it a regular part of your daily routine. Also, you have to remember that you may not be able to do what someone else does; but instead, you do what you can do and find what motivates you to be a more fit version of yourself than you were before. For example, I have disabilities that affect my legs so running isn't something for me so I walk when I can or if I'm having a painful day where walking isn't going to work then I flex and contract my leg muscles (isometrics) to the best of my abilities. The whole idea of that is to still exercise areas of your body to the best of **YOUR ABILITY** and not to neglect them. The Do The Easy Fitness Philosophy is a culture and mindset of exercising to the best of **YOUR ABILITY** whether it's by conventional or alternative means to make YOU a more fit YOU!

DO THE EASY FITNESS

" Weight Loss Motivation: Your Path to a Healthier You"

Welcome to " Weight Loss Motivation: Your Path to a Healthier You", where we'll embark on a journey to help you achieve your weight loss goals in a sensible and sustainable way. No more falling for quick fixes or trendy diets that promise the world but often lead to disappointment. This book is all about providing you with practical advice, real-life strategies, and common sense approaches to help you shed those extra pounds and embrace a healthier lifestyle that lasts.

Chapter 1: Understanding the Basics of Weight Loss

- Simplifying the concept of weight loss: eat less, move more

- How your body uses calories and stores fat
- Busting common weight loss myths
- How to set realistic expectations for your journey

Chapter 2: Setting Achievable Goals and Making a Plan

- Finding your motivation and reasons for wanting to lose weight
- Setting realistic and attainable goals based on your lifestyle
- Keeping track of your progress in a way that works for you
- Creating a practical plan of action to reach your goals

Chapter 3: Eating Well for Weight Loss

- The importance of balanced meals and portion control
- Making healthier food choices without feeling deprived

- Incorporating more fruits, vegetables, and whole foods into your diet
- Practical tips for eating out and managing cravings

Chapter 4: Moving Your Body: Exercise Made Easy

- Discovering enjoyable ways to be active that fit your lifestyle
- Incorporating physical activity into your daily routine
- Practical tips for staying motivated and overcoming exercise barriers
- The benefits of strength training and cardio exercises

Chapter 5: Adopting a Positive Mindset and Healthy Habits

- The power of your mindset in achieving weight loss success
- Building self-confidence and a positive self-image

- Practical strategies for overcoming emotional eating and stress
- Developing healthy habits that support your weight loss journey

Chapter 6: Building a Supportive Environment

- The importance of surrounding yourself with positive influences
- Enlisting the support of friends, family, or weight loss groups
- Finding an accountability partner to stay on track
- Coping with unsupportive environments and staying focused

Chapter 7: Overcoming Challenges and Staying Motivated

- Dealing with weight loss plateaus and overcoming setbacks
- Tips for staying motivated during challenging times

- Handling cravings, emotional hurdles, and negative self-talk
- Common pitfalls to avoid on your weight loss journey

Chapter 8: Maintaining Your Progress and Embracing a Healthy Lifestyle

- Strategies for long-term weight maintenance
- Finding balance and enjoying the process
- Celebrating milestones and non-scale victories
- Incorporating healthy habits into your everyday life

Chapter 1: Understanding the Basics of Weight Loss

Weight loss can sometimes feel like a complex and overwhelming topic. However, at its core, the concept of weight loss can be simplified to a straightforward equation: eat less, move more. In this chapter, we will break down the basics of weight loss, providing you with a clear understanding of the key principles involved.

1.1 Simplifying the concept of weight loss: eat less, move more in a sensible way

Weight loss fundamentally comes down to creating an energy deficit in your body. To shed pounds, you need to consume fewer calories than your body expends. This can be achieved by two main factors: reducing your calorie intake through mindful eating and increasing your calorie expenditure through physical activity.

Eating less involves making conscious choices about the quantity and quality of the food you consume. It's not about starving yourself or following extreme diets. Instead, it's about making healthier food choices, practicing portion control, and listening to your body's hunger and fullness cues.

Moving more involves incorporating regular physical activity into your daily routine. This doesn't mean you have to spend hours at the gym every day. It can be as simple as taking regular walks, engaging in activities you enjoy, or finding ways to be more active throughout your day. The goal is to find ways to increase your overall calorie expenditure and boost your metabolism.

1.2 How your body uses calories and stores fat

Understanding how your body uses calories and stores fat can provide valuable insights into the weight loss process. Calories are the units of energy that your body derives from the food you consume. These calories are utilized for various bodily functions, such as maintaining your metabolism, supporting organ function, and providing energy for physical activity.

When you consume more calories than your body needs for these functions, the excess energy is stored as fat. Fat serves as a reserve fuel source for times when your body requires additional energy. However, if you consistently consume more calories than your body requires, this excess energy accumulates as excess body weight.

Conversely, when you create an energy deficit by consuming fewer calories than your body needs, your body turns to its fat stores to make up for the energy shortfall. This leads to weight loss as the stored fat is utilized for energy.

1.3 Busting common weight loss myths

There are numerous myths and misconceptions surrounding weight loss that can hinder your progress and discourage you from achieving your goals. In this section, we will debunk some of these common weight loss myths:

- Myth 1: Crash diets are the best way to lose weight quickly.
- Myth 2: Certain foods have magical fat-burning properties.
- Myth 3: Carbohydrates are always the enemy when it comes to weight loss.
- Myth 4: Weight loss supplements are a quick and effective solution.
- Myth 5: You have to completely eliminate fats from your diet to lose weight.

By dispelling these myths, you can approach weight loss with a more realistic and informed perspective, focusing on sustainable and healthy strategies that have been proven effective.

1.4 How to set realistic expectations for your journey

One of the keys to successful weight loss is setting realistic expectations from the start. Weight loss is not an overnight process, and it varies from person to person. It's important to understand that sustainable weight loss is gradual and requires patience and persistence.

Instead of fixating on a specific number on the scale, it's essential to focus on overall health and well-being. Set goals that are attainable and sustainable for your body and lifestyle. Celebrate non-scale victories such as increased energy levels, improved fitness, and better overall health markers.

Remember, weight loss is a journey, and there will be ups and downs along the way. By setting realistic expectations and adopting a long-term mindset, you'll be better

Chapter 2: Setting Achievable Goals and Making a Plan

Losing weight successfully starts with setting achievable goals and creating a solid plan. In this chapter, we will explore the key steps involved in setting goals that align with your motivations, tracking your progress effectively, and creating a practical action plan to reach your weight loss objectives.

2.1 Finding your motivation and reasons for wanting to lose weight

Before embarking on your weight loss journey, it's important to dig deep and understand your motivations for wanting to lose weight. What are the reasons behind your desire for change? Are you aiming to improve your overall health and reduce the risk of chronic diseases? Do you want to feel more confident in your body and enhance your self-esteem? Are you seeking to increase your energy levels and improve your quality of life?

Take the time to reflect on these questions and identify your personal motivations. Having a clear understanding of why you want to lose weight will serve as a powerful source of motivation throughout your journey.

2.2 Setting realistic and attainable goals based on your lifestyle

Once you have identified your motivations, it's time to set realistic and attainable goals that are aligned with your lifestyle. It's important to approach goal setting with a sense of realism and practicality. While it's natural to be ambitious, setting goals that are too lofty or unrealistic can set you up for disappointment and frustration.

Consider factors such as your current weight, body composition, health condition, and any physical limitations you may have. Consult with a healthcare professional if needed to ensure that your goals are appropriate for your individual circumstances. Aim for gradual and sustainable weight loss, typically around 1-2 pounds per week, as this is considered a healthy and achievable rate.

Break your larger weight loss goal into smaller milestones that can be celebrated along the way. For example, instead of solely focusing on the final target weight, set smaller goals such as losing 5% of your starting weight or dropping a clothing size. These milestones provide a sense of accomplishment and motivation as you progress on your journey.

2.3 Keeping track of your progress in a way that works for you

Tracking your progress is essential for staying motivated and accountable. Find a tracking method that works for you and aligns with your preferences and lifestyle. Some options include using a journal, mobile apps, spreadsheets, or specialized weight loss platforms. Choose a method that allows you to monitor your food intake, exercise habits, and other relevant factors.

Consider tracking not only your weight but also other measurements and indicators of progress. This can include body measurements (such as waist circumference or body fat percentage), clothing sizes, energy levels, fitness improvements, or even psychological well-being. Non-scale victories are valuable indicators of progress and can help maintain motivation even when the number on the scale fluctuates.

Regularly review your progress and make adjustments as needed. If you notice a plateau or a lack of progress, reassess your approach and consider modifying your plan. Tracking enables you to identify patterns, recognize potential obstacles, and make informed decisions to keep you on track toward your goals.

2.4 Creating a practical plan of action to reach your goals

To turn your goals into reality, you need a practical plan of action. Break down your larger goals into smaller, manageable steps that can be implemented consistently. Consider both nutrition and exercise aspects when creating your plan.

When it comes to nutrition, focus on making healthier food choices and developing balanced eating habits. Incorporate whole, nutrient-dense foods such as fruits, vegetables, lean proteins, whole grains, and healthy fats into your meals. Gradually reduce the consumption of processed foods, sugary beverages, and unhealthy snacks. Practice portion control by being mindful of your serving sizes and paying attention to your body's hunger and fullness cues.

Incorporating regular physical activity is essential for weight loss and overall well-being. Choose activities that you enjoy and that fit into your lifestyle. This can include brisk walking, jogging, cycling, swimming, dancing, or participating in group fitness classes. Aim for a combination of cardiovascular exercise and strength training to maximize the benefits. Start with realistic goals, such as committing to three 30-minute workouts per week, and gradually increase the frequency, duration, and intensity as your fitness level improves.

Consider enlisting support from professionals, such as a registered dietitian or a certified personal trainer, who can provide personalized guidance and help tailor a plan that suits your specific needs and preferences.

Flexibility is key when creating your plan. Life can be unpredictable, and it's important to be adaptable. Accept that there may be occasional deviations or setbacks, and focus on progress rather than perfection. Learn from any challenges or obstacles you encounter and adjust your plan accordingly.

By setting achievable goals and creating a practical plan, you lay a solid foundation for your weight loss journey. Remember to stay committed, embrace the process, and celebrate each milestone along the way. With perseverance, dedication, and a well-thought-out plan, you can achieve your weight loss objectives and improve your overall health and well-being.

Chapter 3: Eating Well for Weight Loss

In Chapter 3, we delve into the crucial aspect of eating well for weight loss. We will explore the importance of balanced meals, portion control, making healthier food choices without feeling deprived, incorporating more fruits, vegetables, and whole foods into your diet, and practical tips for eating out and managing cravings.

3.1 The importance of balanced meals and portion control

Creating balanced meals is key to achieving weight loss goals. By including a variety of food groups, you ensure that your body receives essential nutrients while managing calorie intake. Each meal should ideally contain a combination of lean proteins, whole grains, fruits, vegetables, and healthy fats.

Lean proteins, such as chicken, fish, tofu, or legumes, provide essential amino acids for muscle repair and growth. Whole grains like brown rice, quinoa, and whole wheat bread offer fiber, vitamins, and minerals while keeping you feeling fuller for longer. Fruits and vegetables provide important antioxidants, fiber, and hydration to support overall health. Healthy fats, found in avocados, nuts, and olive oil, help with satiety and provide essential fatty acids.

Portion control is equally important. By being mindful of serving sizes, you can manage your calorie intake effectively. Use measuring cups or a food scale to become familiar with appropriate portion sizes for different types of food. Over time, you'll develop a better understanding of portion sizes, which will help you make informed choices and avoid overeating.

3.2 Making healthier food choices without feeling deprived

Embarking on a weight loss journey does not mean depriving yourself of all the foods you love. It's about finding a balance between nourishing your body and enjoying the foods you enjoy. Here are some strategies to help you make healthier food choices without feeling deprived:

a. Focus on nutrient-dense foods: Fill your plate with nutrient-dense options that provide maximum nutritional value with fewer calories. Choose whole, unprocessed foods over highly processed ones. For example, opt for a colorful salad with a variety of vegetables, grilled chicken breast, and a sprinkle of nuts instead of a calorie-dense, processed meal.

b. Practice mindful eating: Slow down and savor each bite. Pay attention to the taste, texture, and aroma of your food. By eating slowly and mindfully, you allow yourself to fully experience the flavors, which can lead to greater satisfaction with smaller portions. Put away distractions like phones or TVs and focus on the meal in front of you.

c. Allow occasional treats: Deprivation can lead to cravings and ultimately sabotage your weight loss efforts. Allow yourself occasional treats in moderation to satisfy your cravings and prevent feelings of restriction. Enjoy a small piece of dark chocolate or a small portion of your favorite dessert occasionally, savoring each bite and practicing portion control.

d. Discover healthier cooking methods: Experiment with healthier cooking methods that require less oil or fat. Try grilling, baking, steaming, or sautéing with minimal oil instead of deep-frying. These methods can help reduce calorie intake while still providing delicious and flavorful meals.

3.3 Incorporating more fruits, vegetables, and whole foods into your diet

Fruits, vegetables, and whole foods are essential components of a healthy diet and can greatly contribute to weight loss. They are low in calories, high in fiber, and packed with vitamins, minerals, and antioxidants. Here are some tips to help you incorporate more of these nutritious options into your diet:

a. Fill half your plate with vegetables: Make it a habit to include a generous portion of vegetables with every meal. Whether it's leafy greens, colorful bell peppers, crunchy carrots, or roasted Brussels sprouts, the variety of flavors and textures will add excitement to your plate while providing important nutrients.

b. Experiment with new recipes: Explore new ways to prepare fruits and vegetables to keep your meals interesting and enjoyable. Try roasting vegetables with a sprinkle of herbs and spices, blending fruits into smoothies or making homemade fruit salads, or incorporating vegetables into stir-fries or soups. The possibilities are endless.

c. Choose whole grains: Replace refined grains with whole grains to increase your intake of fiber and nutrients. Swap white bread with whole wheat or whole grain bread, opt for brown rice or quinoa instead of white rice, and choose whole grain pasta or oats for added fiber.

d. Snack on whole foods: Instead of reaching for processed snacks, keep a variety of whole foods readily available for snacking. Grab a handful of nuts, enjoy a piece of fresh fruit, or snack on crunchy vegetables with hummus. These options provide nourishment and keep you satisfied between meals.

3.4 Practical tips for eating out and managing cravings

Eating out and managing cravings can present challenges when trying to lose weight. However, with a few strategies in place, you can navigate these situations more successfully:

a. Plan ahead: Before dining out, research the restaurant's menu online and identify healthier options in advance. Look for dishes that are grilled, steamed, or baked, and choose items that are rich in vegetables or lean proteins. Planning ahead helps you make informed choices and resist the temptation of less healthy options.

b. Practice portion control: Restaurants often serve larger portions than what is necessary for a single meal. Consider splitting a dish with a friend or ask for a to-go container at the beginning of the meal, so you can pack up half of your portion to enjoy later. By being mindful of portion sizes, you can enjoy dining out without overeating.

c. Be mindful of sauces and dressings: Many restaurant dishes come with heavy sauces or dressings that can be high in calories. Request dressings, sauces, or condiments on the side, so you have more control over how much you use. Dip your fork into the dressing before taking a bite to enjoy the flavor without overloading on calories.

d. Manage cravings strategically: Cravings are a normal part of the weight loss journey. Instead of giving in to unhealthy options, find healthier alternatives that satisfy your cravings. For example, if you're craving something sweet, try enjoying a piece of fruit or a small serving of Greek yogurt with berries. If you're craving something savory and crunchy, reach for air-popped popcorn or roasted chickpeas.

Remember, achieving weight loss is a journey, and it's important to be patient and kind to yourself along the way. By focusing on balanced meals, portion control, making healthier food choices, and managing cravings, you can establish a sustainable approach to eating well for weight loss.

Chapter 4: Moving Your Body: Exercise Made Easier

In Chapter 4, we delve deeper into the realm of physical activity and explore various aspects of making exercise an enjoyable and integral part of your weight loss journey. We will cover topics such as discovering enjoyable ways to be active that fit your lifestyle, incorporating physical activity into your daily routine, practical tips for staying motivated and overcoming exercise barriers, and the benefits of both strength training and cardio exercises.

4.1 Discovering enjoyable ways to be active that fit your lifestyle

When it comes to exercise, finding activities that you genuinely enjoy is key to staying motivated and consistent. Discovering enjoyable ways to be active can be an exciting and fulfilling journey. Here are some strategies to help you explore and find activities that fit your lifestyle:

a. Explore different activities: Don't be afraid to step out of your comfort zone and try new activities. Sign up for a dance class, join a recreational sports league, or try a martial arts workshop. By experimenting with a variety of activities, you may discover hidden talents and develop a newfound passion for a particular exercise.

b. Incorporate hobbies into exercise: Think about your existing hobbies and find ways to make them more physically active. If you enjoy photography, try going on nature walks or hikes to capture beautiful scenery. If you enjoy gardening, turn it into a full-body workout by incorporating squats, lunges, and digging. By combining exercise with your hobbies, you can make physical activity more enjoyable and seamless.

c. Embrace the great outdoors: Take advantage of the natural surroundings in your area. Go for a jog or bike ride in a nearby park, hike through scenic trails, or try water sports like kayaking or paddleboarding. Exercising in nature not only provides a refreshing change of environment but also offers numerous physical and mental health benefits.

d. Be open to group activities: Joining group activities or fitness classes can add a social element to your exercise routine. It's a great opportunity to meet like-minded individuals, make new friends, and create a supportive community. Consider joining a yoga class, group cycling sessions, or boot camps to experience the camaraderie and motivation that comes with group exercise.

4.2 Incorporating physical activity into your daily routine

Finding time for exercise in a busy schedule can be challenging, but with a little creativity and strategic planning, you can successfully incorporate physical activity into your daily routine. Here are practical tips to help you make exercise a regular part of your day:

a. Prioritize your health: Recognize that exercise is an essential investment in your health and well-being. Make it a priority and allocate dedicated time for physical activity. Consider it as non-negotiable "me time" that benefits both your body and mind.

b. Plan and schedule: Treat exercise like any other important appointment. Set specific workout times in your calendar and stick to them. If you struggle with finding long stretches of time, break your workouts into shorter, more manageable sessions throughout the day. Even 10-15 minutes of exercise can make a positive difference.

c. Make it a family affair: Involve your family members in your exercise routine. Plan outdoor activities, such as family walks or bike rides, that allow everyone to participate and bond while being active. It's a great way to instill healthy habits in your loved ones while enjoying quality time together.

d. Be flexible and adaptable: Life can be unpredictable, and schedules can change at a moment's notice. Be flexible in your approach to exercise and be prepared to adjust your workout plans accordingly. If your original plan falls through, have backup options such as home workouts, online fitness classes, or quick bodyweight routines that you can easily do anywhere.

4.3 Practical tips for staying motivated and overcoming exercise barriers

Staying motivated and overcoming exercise barriers is a common challenge for many individuals. Here are practical tips to help you stay on track and overcome common exercise challenges:

a. Find your why: Understand your personal motivations for wanting to exercise and lose weight. Whether it's to improve your health, boost your energy levels, or set a positive example for your loved ones, knowing your "why" can provide the necessary drive and focus during challenging times.

b. Set realistic goals: Set realistic and achievable goals based on your current fitness level and lifestyle. Break down your long-term goals into smaller, short-term milestones. Celebrate each milestone reached, as this will provide a sense of accomplishment and reinforce your motivation.

c. Track your progress: Keep a record of your exercise activities and track your progress. This can be done through a workout journal, a fitness app, or a simple calendar. Seeing your progress visually can be highly motivating and help you stay accountable to your fitness goals.

d. Mix it up: Avoid getting stuck in a monotonous exercise routine by incorporating variety into your workouts. Try different types of exercises, alternate between indoor and outdoor activities, or participate in seasonal sports. By keeping your workouts fresh and exciting, you'll be more likely to stay engaged and motivated.

e. Seek support: Surround yourself with a supportive network of friends, family, or like-minded individuals who share your fitness goals. Engage in positive conversations, share your challenges and victories, and seek support when needed. Having a support system can provide encouragement, accountability, and a sense of camaraderie.

f. Overcome mental barriers: Often, the biggest barriers to exercise are mental rather than physical. Address negative self-talk, self-doubt, or limiting beliefs that may be holding you back. Remind yourself of the progress you've made and the positive changes you've experienced. Practice self-compassion and focus on the joy and satisfaction that comes from being active.

4.4 The benefits of strength training and cardio exercises

Understanding the benefits of both strength training and cardio exercises can motivate you to incorporate them into your routine. Here are the advantages of each:

a. Strength training: Strength training exercises offer numerous benefits for weight loss and overall health. By engaging in activities such as weightlifting, resistance training, or bodyweight exercises, you can experience the following advantages:

- Increased muscle mass: Strength training helps build lean muscle mass, which contributes to a higher metabolic rate. This means you burn more calories even at rest, aiding in weight loss and weight maintenance.
- Improved body composition: Building muscle and reducing body fat through strength training can lead to a more toned and defined physique.

- Enhanced bone density: Strength training helps improve bone mineral density, reducing the risk of osteoporosis and promoting long-term bone health.
- Enhanced functional fitness: Strengthening your muscles and improving muscular endurance makes daily activities easier and reduces the risk of injury.
- Increased metabolism: Muscle tissue is metabolically active, meaning it burns more calories than fat tissue. By increasing muscle mass through strength training, you can boost your metabolism and support weight loss efforts.

b. Cardio exercises: Cardiovascular exercises, often known as aerobic exercises, offer numerous benefits for weight loss and overall fitness. Engaging in activities such as running, cycling, swimming, or dancing can provide the following advantages:

- Increased calorie burn: Cardio exercises elevate your heart rate, which helps burn calories and support weight loss.
- Improved cardiovascular health: Regular cardio exercise strengthens your heart, improves blood circulation, and enhances cardiovascular fitness. This can reduce the risk of heart disease, stroke, and other cardiovascular conditions.
- Increased endurance: Cardio exercises improve your body's ability to utilize oxygen efficiently, leading to improved stamina and endurance. This allows you to engage in physical activities for longer periods without feeling fatigued.
- Elevated mood and reduced stress: Cardio exercises stimulate the release of endorphins, which are natural mood-boosting hormones. Regular cardio workouts can help reduce

stress, anxiety, and symptoms of depression.
- Improved lung capacity: Cardio exercises challenge your respiratory system, leading to increased lung capacity and improved respiratory function.

To create a well-rounded exercise routine, aim to include both strength training and cardio exercises. Start with two to three days of strength training per week, targeting all major muscle groups. Supplement it with cardiovascular activities on most days of the week, gradually increasing intensity and duration as your fitness improves.

By discovering enjoyable ways to be active, incorporating physical activity into your daily routine, staying motivated, and recognizing the benefits of strength training and cardio exercises, you can make exercise an integral part of your weight loss journey.

Remember, finding activities you love and creating a sustainable exercise routine will not only help you achieve your weight loss goals but also enhance your overall well-being.

Chapter 5: Adopting a Positive Mindset and Healthy Habits

In Chapter 5, let's talk about the crucial role of mindset and habits in achieving weight loss success. We explore the power of a positive mindset, building self-confidence and a positive self-image, practical strategies for overcoming emotional eating and stress, and the importance of developing healthy habits that support your weight loss journey.

5.1 The power of your mindset in achieving weight loss success

Your mindset plays a significant role in your weight loss journey. By cultivating a positive and resilient mindset, you can overcome challenges, stay motivated, and ultimately achieve success. Here are some key aspects to consider:

a. Believe in yourself: Develop a strong belief in your ability to succeed. Embrace a growth mindset, understanding that weight loss is a journey of learning and progress. Believe that you have the capacity to make lasting changes and achieve your goals.

b. Focus on progress, not perfection: Weight loss is not a linear process, and setbacks are inevitable. Instead of fixating on perfection, shift your focus to progress. Celebrate each small step forward, whether it's making healthier food choices, completing a workout, or overcoming a personal challenge. Recognize that every effort counts and contributes to your overall progress.

c. Practice self-compassion: Be kind and forgiving to yourself throughout your weight loss journey. Acknowledge that setbacks and mistakes are a natural part of the process. Treat yourself with the same kindness and understanding that you would extend to a friend who is on a similar journey.

d. Visualize your success: Take a moment each day to visualize yourself achieving your weight loss goals. Imagine how you will look, feel, and move with a healthier body. Visualization can help reinforce your motivation and create a positive outlook.

e. Surround yourself with positivity: Surround yourself with positive influences and supportive individuals who uplift and inspire you. Seek out communities, whether online or in-person, that share similar goals and provide encouragement. Limit exposure to negative or judgmental influences that may undermine your self-confidence.

5.2 Building self-confidence and a positive self-image

Building self-confidence and nurturing a positive self-image are essential components of a successful weight loss journey. Here are some strategies to help boost your self-confidence:

a. Celebrate non-scale victories: Instead of solely focusing on the number on the scale, celebrate the non-scale victories along the way. These can include improved energy levels, increased strength, better sleep quality, or fitting into clothes that were previously too tight. Recognize and appreciate the positive changes happening in your body and overall well-being.

b. Practice positive self-talk: Be mindful of your internal dialogue and replace negative self-talk with positive affirmations. Instead of criticizing yourself for setbacks or perceived shortcomings, remind yourself of your strengths, achievements, and the progress you have made. Use positive statements to uplift and encourage yourself throughout the journey.

c. Set realistic expectations: Set realistic expectations for your weight loss journey. Understand that sustainable weight loss takes time and effort. Avoid comparing yourself to others or striving for an unrealistic ideal. Embrace your unique journey and focus on becoming the best version of yourself.

d. Emphasize your strengths: Identify your strengths and leverage them to support your weight loss efforts. Whether it's your determination, discipline, or ability to adapt, acknowledge and utilize these strengths to overcome challenges and stay motivated.

e. Practice self-care: Take care of your physical, mental, and emotional well-being. Prioritize activities that nourish your body and soul, such as getting enough sleep, practicing relaxation techniques, engaging in hobbies you enjoy, and spending time with loved ones. When you prioritize self-care, you enhance your overall sense of well-being, which positively impacts your self-confidence.

5.3 Practical strategies for overcoming emotional eating and stress

Emotional eating and stress can often hinder weight loss progress. However, by adopting practical strategies, you can overcome these challenges and develop healthier coping mechanisms. Here are some strategies to consider:

a. Identify triggers: Become aware of the situations, emotions, or events that trigger emotional eating or stress. Keep a journal to track patterns and identify common triggers. This self-awareness will help you develop alternative strategies to manage those triggers effectively.

b. Seek alternative outlets: Find alternative activities or outlets to channel your emotions or cope with stress. Engage in activities that bring you joy, such as listening to music, practicing art, writing in a journal, or engaging in physical activity. These activities can help you manage stress and emotions without resorting to food as a coping mechanism.

c. Develop a support system: Surround yourself with a strong support system that understands your weight loss journey and can provide emotional support during challenging times. This can include family, friends, or even joining a support group where you can share experiences, exchange advice, and receive encouragement.

d. Practice mindful eating: Mindful eating involves being fully present and aware of your food choices and eating habits. Pay attention to your hunger and fullness cues, savor each bite, and eat without distractions. This practice allows you to develop a healthier relationship with food, understand your body's signals, and make conscious choices that align with your weight loss goals.

e. Implement stress-management techniques: Stress can often trigger emotional eating or disrupt your weight loss efforts. Explore stress-management techniques such as deep breathing exercises, yoga, or engaging in regular physical activity to reduce stress levels. Additionally, prioritize self-care activities such as getting enough sleep, practicing relaxation techniques, and finding time for activities that bring you joy and relaxation.

5.4 Developing healthy habits that support your weight loss journey

Developing healthy habits is crucial for sustainable weight loss and long-term success. Here are practical strategies to help you establish healthy habits:

a. Set realistic and achievable goals: Break down your weight loss goals into smaller, manageable steps. Set specific and achievable goals that align with your lifestyle and priorities. This approach allows you to build momentum and celebrate regular achievements, reinforcing the development of healthy habits.

b. Create a routine: Establishing a consistent routine can help you integrate healthy habits seamlessly into your daily life. Plan regular meal times, set aside dedicated time for physical activity, and prioritize self-care activities. Consistency in your routine creates a sense of structure and makes it easier to stick to your healthy habits.

c. Prioritize nutrition: Focus on nourishing your body with whole, nutrient-dense foods. Make gradual changes to your eating habits, such as incorporating more fruits, vegetables, lean proteins, and whole grains into your meals. Aim for balanced and portion-controlled meals that provide sustained energy and support your weight loss goals.

d. Practice mindful portion control: Pay attention to portion sizes and be mindful of your body's hunger and fullness cues. Use smaller plates, bowls, and utensils to visually create the perception of a satisfying meal. Slow down your eating pace, savor each bite, and listen to your body's signals to prevent overeating.

e. Stay hydrated: Drinking an adequate amount of water is essential for overall health and weight loss. Ensure you stay hydrated throughout the day by carrying a water bottle with you and making it a habit to drink water regularly. Water not only supports your body's functions but also helps curb hunger and cravings.

f. Get enough sleep: Adequate sleep is vital for weight management and overall well-being. Aim for a consistent sleep schedule and prioritize getting 7-9 hours of quality sleep each night. Establish a relaxing bedtime routine and create a sleep-friendly environment to optimize your sleep quality.

g. Practice stress management: Chronic stress can disrupt your weight loss efforts. Prioritize stress management techniques such as regular exercise, meditation, deep breathing exercises, or engaging in activities that bring you joy and relaxation. By managing stress effectively, you can reduce the likelihood of turning to food for comfort.

By adopting a positive mindset, building self-confidence, implementing strategies for overcoming emotional eating and stress, and developing healthy habits, you create a solid foundation for your weight loss journey. Remember that small, consistent changes over time lead to significant results. Embrace the process, be patient with yourself, and celebrate each step forward.

Chapter 6: Building a Supportive Environment

In Chapter 6, we explore the significance of creating a supportive environment that nurtures your weight loss journey. We delve into the importance of surrounding yourself with positive influences, enlisting the support of friends, family, or weight loss groups, finding an accountability partner to stay on track, and strategies for coping with unsupportive environments while staying focused on your goals.

6.1 The importance of surrounding yourself with positive influences

When it comes to weight loss, the company you keep can greatly impact your success. Surrounding yourself with positive influences creates an atmosphere that nurtures healthy habits and reinforces positive choices. Here are additional reasons why a positive environment matters:

a. Energy and enthusiasm: Positive influences radiate energy and enthusiasm, which can be contagious. Being around individuals who are optimistic, passionate, and dedicated to their own well-being can inspire you to stay motivated and committed to your weight loss journey.

b. Knowledge sharing: A positive environment encourages knowledge sharing. When you surround yourself with like-minded individuals, you have the opportunity to learn from their experiences, gather insights, and discover new strategies that can help you overcome challenges and achieve your goals more effectively.

c. Constructive feedback and advice: Positive influences provide constructive feedback and advice when necessary. They can offer a fresh perspective, identify areas for improvement, and suggest alternative approaches to help you overcome obstacles. Their supportive guidance can keep you on the right track and help you make informed decisions.

d. Emotional support and understanding: Having a supportive environment means having people who understand the emotional aspects of your weight loss journey. They can empathize with your struggles, offer words of encouragement, and provide a safe space for you to share your feelings and experiences. This emotional support is invaluable during challenging times.

6.2 Enlisting the support of friends, family, or weight loss groups

Enlisting the support of friends, family, or joining weight loss groups can provide a strong support system that can enhance your weight loss journey. Here are additional considerations for seeking support:

a. Accountability and commitment: When you involve others in your weight loss journey, you gain a sense of accountability. Knowing that someone is invested in your success can motivate you to stay committed to your goals. Sharing your progress with others and having them cheer you on creates a sense of responsibility to yourself and those supporting you.

b. Encouragement and motivation: Friends, family, or weight loss groups can provide continuous encouragement and motivation. They can celebrate your achievements, offer words of encouragement during setbacks, and remind you of your progress when you may feel discouraged. Their unwavering support can keep your spirits high and your focus on track.

c. Practical tips and experiences: Those who have already gone through a weight loss journey can offer practical tips, insights, and advice based on their experiences. They can share strategies that worked for them, provide recommendations for healthy recipes or workout routines, and offer guidance on how to overcome common obstacles. This shared knowledge can save you time, effort, and trial-and-error.

d. Social connections and camaraderie: Enlisting support from friends, family, or weight loss groups can foster social connections and a sense of camaraderie. Engaging with others who are on a similar journey creates a community where you can share successes, discuss challenges, and find understanding and validation. The sense of belonging can boost your motivation and make your weight loss journey more enjoyable.

6.3 Finding an accountability partner to stay on track

An accountability partner can play a crucial role in keeping you focused and accountable on your weight loss journey. Here are additional insights on finding an accountability partner:

a. Shared goals and values: Look for an accountability partner who shares similar goals and values regarding health and well-being. When you have common ground, your partner can better understand your aspirations, provide relevant support, and hold you accountable based on shared principles.

b. Regular check-ins and progress tracking: Establish a routine for regular check-ins and progress tracking with your accountability partner. This can be done weekly, biweekly, or monthly, depending on your preferences and goals. During these check-ins, you can discuss your progress, challenges, and set new milestones. Tracking your progress together ensures that you stay accountable and continue moving forward.

c. Open and honest communication: A successful accountability partnership requires open and honest communication. Both partners should feel comfortable sharing their struggles, setbacks, and victories. This transparency allows for constructive feedback, encouragement, and problem-solving. It's important to establish an environment of trust and mutual respect.

d. Mutual support and motivation: An accountability partnership is a two-way street. Both partners should be committed to supporting and motivating each other. Celebrate each other's successes, provide encouragement during challenging times, and offer suggestions or solutions when needed. The partnership thrives on reciprocity and a shared commitment to growth and progress.

e. Flexibility and adaptability: Recognize that circumstances may change, and flexibility is key to maintaining a successful accountability partnership. Life can present unexpected challenges or interruptions, but with open communication and flexibility, you can adjust your check-in schedule or modify your approach while still supporting each other's goals.

6.4 Coping with unsupportive environments and staying focused

Unfortunately, not all environments are conducive to weight loss. However, with determination and resilience, you can navigate unsupportive environments and stay focused on your goals. Consider the following strategies:

a. Seek understanding and educate others: Communicate your needs and weight loss goals to those in your unsupportive environment. Share your motivations, explain the benefits of your journey, and help them understand how their support can positively impact your progress. Providing information and educating others about the importance of your goals can foster understanding and potentially garner support.

b. Lead by example: Sometimes, the best way to influence an unsupportive environment is to lead by example. Show the positive changes you're making in your own life through healthy eating choices, regular exercise, and a positive mindset. When others witness the positive impact on your well-being and see your dedication, they may become more supportive and inspired to make changes themselves.

c. Seek external support: If your immediate environment remains unsupportive, seek support from external sources. Join online communities or forums where you can connect with individuals who are on a similar journey. These communities provide a virtual support system, where you can share experiences, receive advice, and find encouragement from like-minded individuals.

d. Focus on your own well-being: When faced with an unsupportive environment, prioritize your own well-being and focus on your goals. Remind yourself of the reasons why you embarked on this weight loss journey and the positive impact it has on your life. Stay committed to your own growth and development, and do not let external influences derail your progress.

e. Seek professional guidance: If coping with an unsupportive environment becomes overwhelming, consider seeking professional guidance from a therapist, counselor, or weight loss coach. These professionals can provide you with strategies to navigate challenging situations, cope with negative influences, and help you stay focused on your goals.

Remember, your weight loss journey is ultimately about taking care of yourself, improving your health, and embracing a positive lifestyle. While a supportive environment can greatly enhance your progress, staying focused and committed to your goals regardless of external influences is key. With determination, resilience, and the right support system, you can navigate any challenges that come your way and achieve long-term success.

Chapter 7: Overcoming Challenges and Staying Motivated

In chapter 7, we deal with Overcoming Challenges and Staying Motivated. Weight loss plateaus and setbacks are common on any weight loss journey. They can be frustrating and demotivating, but with the right strategies, you can overcome them and continue making progress. Here are additional insights on dealing with plateaus and setbacks:

7.1 Dealing with weight loss plateaus and overcoming setbacks

a. Assess your approach: When faced with a weight loss plateau or setback, it's essential to assess your approach. Reflect on your eating habits, exercise routine, and overall lifestyle. Consider whether any factors might be hindering your progress. Are you consuming hidden calories or not pushing yourself enough during workouts? By identifying areas for improvement, you can make necessary adjustments and reignite your progress.

b. Seek professional advice: If you're struggling to break through a plateau or overcome setbacks, consider seeking guidance from professionals such as registered dietitians, personal trainers, or weight loss coaches. These experts can provide personalized insights, tailor-made plans, and expert advice to help you overcome challenges and optimize your weight loss journey.

c. Practice patience and resilience: Weight loss plateaus and setbacks are normal parts of the journey. It's crucial to remain patient and resilient during these times. Understand that your body might need time to readjust, and setbacks are opportunities for learning and growth. Trust the process, stay committed to your goals, and remember that sustainable weight loss is a marathon, not a sprint.

d. Review and adjust your goals: If you find yourself continuously facing plateaus or setbacks, it may be beneficial to review and adjust your goals. Ensure that they are realistic, attainable, and aligned with your current lifestyle and circumstances. By setting achievable milestones, you can experience regular victories, maintain motivation, and stay on track.

e. Celebrate non-scale victories: Instead of solely focusing on the number on the scale, celebrate non-scale victories. These victories can include improved energy levels, increased strength and endurance, better sleep quality, or enhanced overall well-being. Recognizing and celebrating these achievements will boost your motivation and reinforce the positive changes you're making.

7.2 Tips for staying motivated during challenging times

a. Find your deeper motivation: Discovering and understanding your deeper motivations for losing weight is crucial for staying motivated during challenging times. Reflect on the reasons behind your weight loss journey. Is it to improve your health, gain confidence, set an example for your loved ones, or enhance your quality of life? Connecting with your inner motivations will provide a strong foundation for your motivation.

b. Visualize your success: Visualization is a powerful tool for staying motivated. Take a few moments each day to visualize yourself successfully achieving your weight loss goals. Picture how you will feel, look, and live your life when you reach your desired weight. This mental imagery will inspire and fuel your motivation, keeping you focused on the positive outcomes.

c. Find accountability partners: Engage with like-minded individuals who are also on a weight loss journey. Join support groups, online communities, or fitness classes where you can connect with others facing similar challenges. Sharing experiences, progress, and setbacks with accountability partners will create a supportive network that keeps you motivated, inspired, and accountable.

d. Set rewards and incentives: Establish a system of rewards and incentives for reaching specific milestones or achieving your goals. Treat yourself to non-food rewards such as a spa day, new workout gear, a weekend getaway, or a new book. Having something to look forward to can boost your motivation and make the journey more enjoyable.

e. Journal your progress: Maintain a weight loss journal to track your progress, thoughts, and emotions. Write down your goals, daily achievements, and any setbacks you encounter. Reflecting on your journey through journaling allows you to see how far you've come, identify patterns or triggers, and celebrate the small wins. It's a tangible reminder of your dedication and progress, keeping you motivated and focused.

7.3 Handling cravings, emotional hurdles, and negative self-talk

a. Distinguish between hunger and emotions: Cravings and emotional eating often stem from emotions rather than actual hunger. Practice mindfulness to distinguish between physical hunger and emotional triggers. Before reaching for food, ask yourself if you're genuinely hungry or if there's an underlying emotional need. Find alternative ways to address your emotions, such as talking to a friend, engaging in a hobby, or practicing relaxation techniques.

b. Create a supportive environment:
Surround yourself with a supportive
environment that promotes healthy choices
and discourages emotional eating. Stock
your pantry with nutritious foods, remove
tempting snacks, and fill your refrigerator
with fresh fruits and vegetables. Surround
yourself with positive influences who
encourage and support your weight loss
goals.

c. Develop healthy coping mechanisms:
Instead of turning to food as a coping
mechanism, find alternative strategies to
manage stress, boredom, or sadness.
Engage in activities that bring you joy, such
as exercising, practicing yoga, listening to
music, or pursuing a creative hobby.
Developing healthy coping mechanisms will
help you navigate emotional hurdles
without relying on food.

d. Challenge negative self-talk: Negative
self-talk can be detrimental to your

motivation and self-esteem. Whenever negative thoughts arise, consciously challenge them with positive affirmations. Remind yourself of your progress, strengths, and the efforts you're making to achieve your goals. Surround yourself with positive influences and practice self-compassion. Treat yourself with kindness and understanding throughout your journey.

e. Seek professional support: If emotional hurdles, cravings, or negative self-talk persist, consider seeking professional support. A therapist, counselor, or psychologist can provide valuable guidance, helping you address emotional barriers, develop healthier coping mechanisms, and cultivate a positive mindset.

By implementing these strategies, you'll be better equipped to overcome challenges, stay motivated, and maintain a positive mindset throughout your weight loss journey. Remember, your journey is unique, and it's important to focus on progress rather than perfection. Embrace the process, learn from setbacks, and celebrate every step forward toward your ultimate weight loss goals.

Chapter 8: Maintaining Your Progress and Embracing a Healthy Lifestyle

Welcome to Chapter 8: Maintaining Your Progress and Embracing a Healthy Lifestyle. Congratulations on reaching this stage of your weight loss journey! By now, you have achieved significant results and made incredible strides towards a healthier and happier version of yourself. However, the journey does not end here. In this chapter, we will explore essential strategies and practices to help you sustain your progress, cultivate a positive mindset, and fully embrace a healthy lifestyle for the long term. Maintaining your weight loss and embracing a healthy lifestyle is about more than just numbers on a scale—it is a holistic approach that encompasses nourishing your body, nurturing your mind, and creating sustainable habits. Let us talk about the key principles and actionable steps that will empower you to continue your transformation and thrive in your newfound health and well-being.

8.1 Strategies for long-term weight maintenance

a. Gradual transition: Transitioning from a weight loss phase to weight maintenance requires a gradual approach. Slowly increase your calorie intake to match your energy needs without causing weight gain. Gradual adjustments allow your body to adapt, minimizing the chances of rebound weight gain.

b. Consistency is key: Maintaining weight loss requires consistency in your eating habits and exercise routine. Stick to the healthy habits you've developed during your weight loss journey, such as balanced meals, portion control, and regular physical activity. Consistency ensures that you continue to make progress and prevents the return of old habits.

c. Regular monitoring: Regularly monitor your weight and body measurements to stay aware of any changes. It's normal for your weight to fluctuate slightly, but keep an eye on any significant shifts. If you notice a consistent upward trend, adjust your habits accordingly to prevent further weight gain.

d. Mindful eating: Continue practicing mindful eating even after achieving your weight loss goals. Pay attention to your hunger and fullness cues, savor the flavors and textures of your food, and eat slowly. Mindful eating helps you maintain a healthy relationship with food, prevent overeating, and enjoy your meals without guilt.

e. Stay active: Physical activity remains crucial for weight maintenance. Aim for at least 150 minutes of moderate-intensity aerobic activity per week, along with strength training exercises. Find activities you enjoy to keep yourself motivated and engaged. Remember that exercise is not just for weight control but also for overall health and well-being.

8.2 Finding balance and enjoying the process

a. Flexible approach: Embrace a flexible approach to your healthy lifestyle. Allow yourself occasional indulgences or treats without guilt. Allowing room for flexibility and enjoyment helps prevent feelings of deprivation and promotes a sustainable relationship with food.

b. Enjoyable activities: Engage in physical activities that you genuinely enjoy. Explore various options such as hiking, dancing, swimming, or team sports. By finding pleasure in your workouts, you'll be more likely to maintain an active lifestyle in the long run.

c. Social support: Seek out social support to enhance your enjoyment of a healthy lifestyle. Exercise with friends, join fitness classes together, or participate in group activities. Having a social support system fosters a sense of community and makes healthy living more enjoyable.

d. Mind-body practices: Incorporate mind-body practices like yoga, meditation, or tai chi into your routine. These practices help reduce stress, improve mental well-being, and create a sense of balance and harmony in your life.

8.3 Celebrating milestones and non-scale victories

a. Set new goals: Celebrate reaching your initial weight loss goals by setting new ones. These goals can be related to improving fitness, achieving specific exercise milestones, or trying new activities. By continuously setting and achieving goals, you stay motivated and engaged in your healthy lifestyle journey.

b. Non-scale victories: Shift your focus from solely relying on the scale and celebrate non-scale victories. These victories can include improved energy levels, better sleep quality, increased strength and endurance, improved mood, or fitting into smaller clothing sizes. Recognizing and celebrating these achievements reinforces your progress and keeps you motivated.

c. Reward yourself: Acknowledge your hard work and dedication by rewarding yourself with non-food treats when you achieve milestones or reach specific goals. Treat yourself to a massage, a new workout outfit, a spa day, or a weekend getaway. These rewards serve as positive reinforcement for your efforts and further motivate you to maintain your progress.

8.4 Incorporating healthy habits into your everyday life

a. Meal planning and preparation: Continue practicing meal planning and preparation to ensure you have nutritious meals readily available. Plan your meals for the week, create a shopping list, and dedicate time for meal prep. Having healthy meals on hand saves time, reduces the temptation for unhealthy choices, and supports your long-term weight maintenance.

b. Prioritize self-care: Make self-care a priority in your daily routine. Set aside time for activities that promote relaxation, reduce stress, and improve your overall well-being. This can include activities like taking a bath, practicing mindfulness, reading a book, or engaging in a hobby. Prioritizing self-care helps you maintain a healthy balance and prevents burnout.

c. Regular check-ins: Schedule regular check-ins with yourself to assess your progress, reassess goals, and make adjustments as needed. Reflect on your habits, identify areas for improvement, and celebrate your successes. Regular check-ins help you stay accountable, maintain focus, and make necessary changes to support your ongoing healthy lifestyle.

8.5 Building a support system for long-term success

a. Engage with your community: Stay connected with like-minded individuals who are also on a journey towards a healthy lifestyle. Join fitness classes, wellness groups, or online communities where you can share experiences, exchange tips, and provide support to one another. Building a support system fosters motivation, accountability, and a sense of camaraderie.

b. Family involvement: Involve your family members in your healthy lifestyle journey. Encourage them to join you in nutritious meal planning, cooking, and physical activities. Creating a supportive environment at home helps maintain healthy habits for everyone and strengthens family bonds.

c. Professional support: Consider seeking ongoing professional support to ensure long-term success. A registered dietitian, personal trainer, or health coach can provide guidance, monitor your progress, and help you navigate challenges that may arise along the way. They can offer personalized advice, tailored meal plans, and exercise programs to support your specific needs.

d. Continuing education: Stay informed about the latest research, trends, and developments in nutrition and fitness. Read books, attend seminars or workshops, and follow reputable health and wellness websites to expand your knowledge. Continuing education empowers you to make informed choices and adapt your healthy lifestyle as new information emerges.

e. Practice self-compassion: Remember to be kind to yourself throughout your journey. Embrace the ups and downs, acknowledge that setbacks may occur, and practice self-compassion during challenging times. Treat yourself with understanding and forgiveness, and use setbacks as opportunities for growth and learning.

8.6 Finding enjoyment in new activities

a. Exploring new recipes: Expand your culinary repertoire by trying new healthy recipes. Explore different cuisines, experiment with unique ingredients, and challenge yourself to cook meals that are both nutritious and delicious. Engaging in the creative process of cooking can be enjoyable and help you discover new favorite dishes.

b. Outdoor activities: Take advantage of the great outdoors and engage in activities that allow you to stay active while enjoying nature. Go for hikes, bike rides, or walks in the park. Try activities like gardening, kayaking, or playing a sport with friends. Outdoor activities provide a refreshing change of scenery and help you stay connected with nature.

c. Group fitness classes: Join group fitness classes to add variety and social interaction to your exercise routine. From dance classes to boot camps, there is a wide range of options available that cater to different interests and fitness levels. Exercising in a group setting can be motivating, fun, and an opportunity to meet new people with similar goals.

d. Mindful movement practices: Explore alternative mindful movement practices such as Pilates, barre, or low-impact aerobics. These practices not only improve strength, flexibility, and balance but also help cultivate mindfulness, body awareness, and a sense of accomplishment. Find a practice that resonates with you and brings joy to your fitness routine.

8.7 Nurturing self-care and self-compassion

a. Relaxation techniques: Incorporate relaxation techniques into your daily routine to reduce stress and promote self-care. Explore practices such as deep breathing exercises, progressive muscle relaxation, or guided imagery. These techniques can help you unwind, reduce tension, and restore a sense of calm amidst the demands of daily life.

b. Pampering rituals: Treat yourself to regular pampering rituals that promote self-care and enhance your well-being. Set aside time for activities like taking a soothing bath, getting a massage, or indulging in a facial or spa treatment. These rituals provide an opportunity to relax, rejuvenate, and prioritize your own needs.

c. Mindful self-reflection: Engage in regular moments of self-reflection to check in with yourself and cultivate self-awareness. Take time to journal, meditate, or simply sit in quiet contemplation. Reflect on your progress, achievements, and areas for growth. Practice self-compassion by acknowledging your efforts and celebrating even the smallest victories.

d. Prioritizing leisure activities: Carve out time for activities that bring you joy and relaxation. Engage in hobbies, interests, or creative pursuits that allow you to unwind and express yourself. Whether it's painting, playing a musical instrument, engaging in crafts, or exploring new hobbies, dedicating time to leisure activities nourishes your soul and supports your overall well-being.

8.8 Embracing a lifelong commitment

a. Emphasizing health over weight: Shift your focus from solely weight-related goals to a broader emphasis on overall health and well-being. Place importance on nourishing your body with wholesome foods, engaging in regular physical activity, and prioritizing self-care. Recognize that health encompasses more than a number on the scale and is a lifelong journey.

b. Celebrating progress and milestones: Continue celebrating your progress and milestones along the way. Take time to acknowledge and appreciate how far you've come, whether it's reaching a fitness milestone, overcoming a specific challenge, or maintaining your weight loss over a significant period. Celebrating your achievements reinforces your commitment and motivates you to keep striving for a healthy lifestyle.

c. Flexibility and adaptation: Understand that life is filled with changes and challenges, and your healthy lifestyle should be adaptable to different circumstances. Embrace flexibility in your approach, being willing to adjust your routines and habits as needed. Learn to navigate obstacles and find creative solutions to maintain your progress and continue embracing a healthy lifestyle.

d. Continued learning and growth: Stay curious and committed to learning about nutrition, fitness, and overall well-being. Keep yourself informed about the latest research, trends, and strategies that can enhance your healthy lifestyle journey. Explore new resources, attend workshops or seminars, and seek guidance from professionals to expand your knowledge and refine your approach.

By incorporating these strategies into your everyday life and nurturing a strong support system, you will not only maintain your weight loss progress but also continue to embrace a healthy and fulfilling lifestyle for years to come. Embrace the journey, stay committed, and celebrate the positive impact your healthy habits have on your overall well-being.

Congratulations on completing **DO THE EASY FITNESS " Weight Loss Motivation: Your Path to a Healthier You"** and taking the first step toward a healthier you. Remember, this journey is about making sensible choices, creating sustainable habits, and embracing a lifestyle that supports your well-being. By implementing the practical advice and strategies provided in this book, you're equipped to achieve your weight loss goals and maintain your progress in the long run. Get ready to unlock your full potential, transform your life, and enjoy the benefits of a healthier and happier you. **THANK YOU FOR THE SUPPORT AND FOR MAKING THE CHOICE FOR A BETTER YOU!!!!!!**